Symptom Tracker

Date	Symptoms	Severity	Possible Triggers	Actions Taken

Symptom Tracker

Date	Symptoms	Severity	Possible Triggers	Actions Taken

Symptom Tracker

Date	Symptoms	Severity	Possible Triggers	Actions Taken

Symptom Tracker

Date	Symptoms	Severity	Possible Triggers	Actions Taken

Symptom Tracker

Date	Symptoms	Severity	Possible Triggers	Actions Taken

Symptom Tracker

Date	Symptoms	Severity	Possible Triggers	Actions Taken

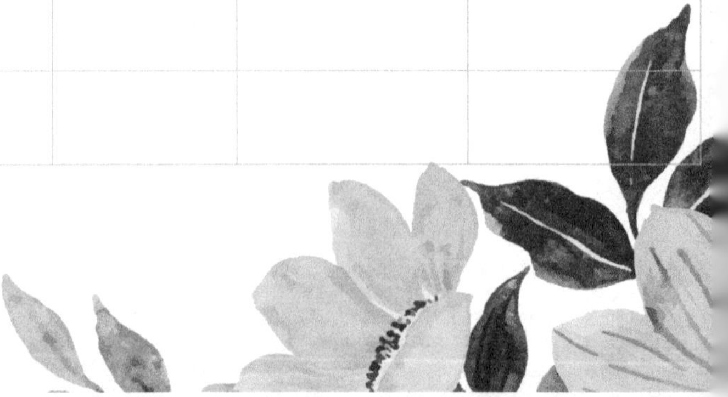

Symptom Tracker

Date	Symptoms	Severity	Possible Triggers	Actions Taken

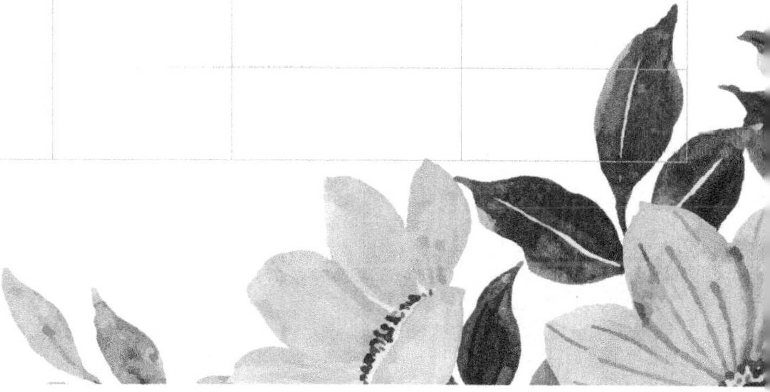

Symptom Tracker

Date	Symptoms	Severity	Possible Triggers	Actions Taken

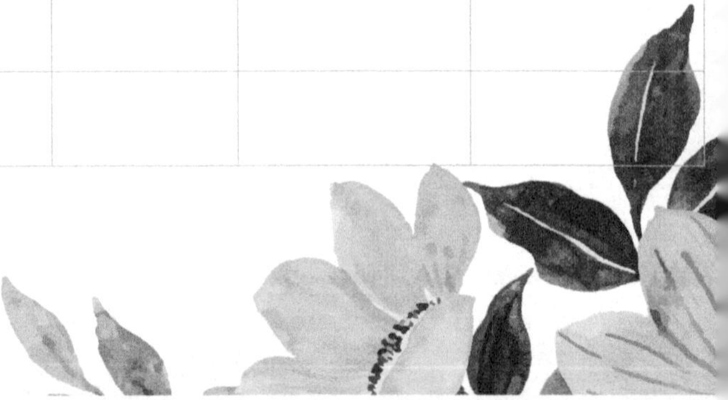

Symptom Tracker

Date	Symptoms	Severity	Possible Triggers	Actions Taken

Symptom Tracker

Date	Symptoms	Severity	Possible Triggers	Actions Taken

Symptom Tracker

Date	Symptoms	Severity	Possible Triggers	Actions Taken

Symptom Tracker

Date	Symptoms	Severity	Possible Triggers	Actions Taken

Symptom Tracker

Date	Symptoms	Severity	Possible Triggers	Actions Taken

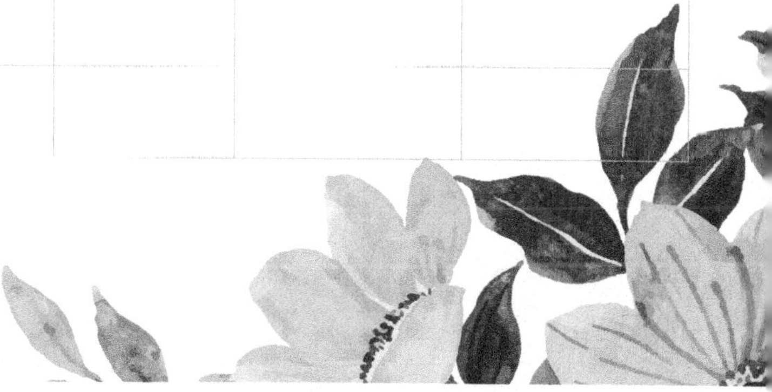

Symptom Tracker

Date	Symptoms	Severity	Possible Triggers	Actions Taken

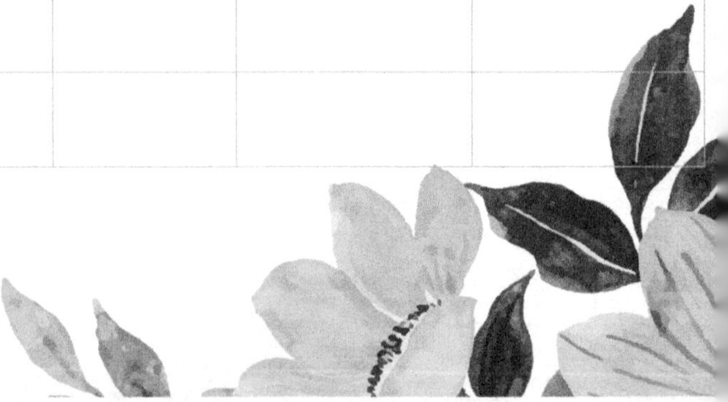

Symptom Tracker

Date	Symptoms	Severity	Possible Triggers	Actions Taken

Symptom Tracker

Date	Symptoms	Severity	Possible Triggers	Actions Taken

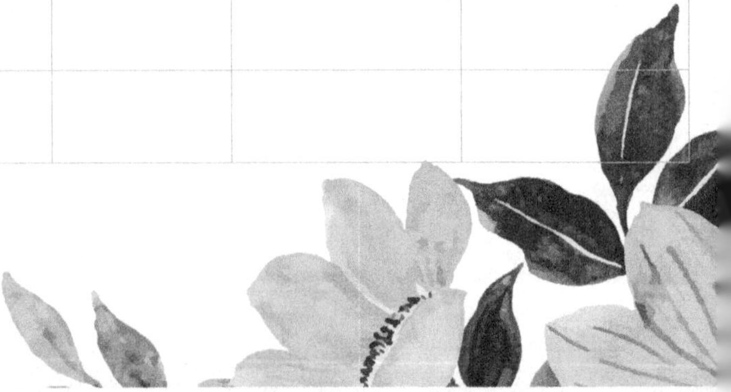

Symptom Tracker

Date	Symptoms	Severity	Possible Triggers	Actions Taken

Symptom Tracker

Date	Symptoms	Severity	Possible Triggers	Actions Taken

Symptom Tracker

Date	Symptoms	Severity	Possible Triggers	Actions Taken

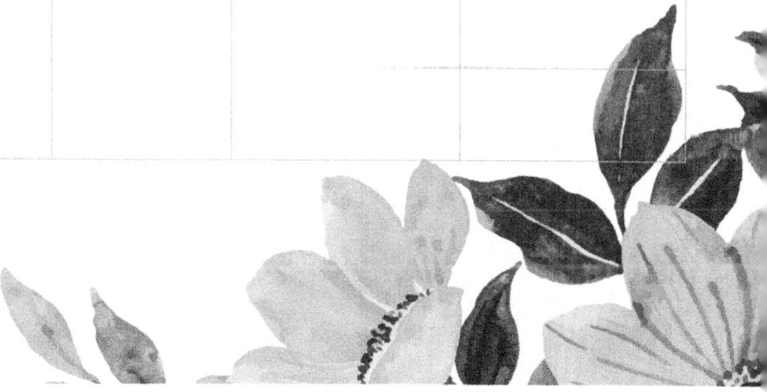

Symptom Tracker

Date	Symptoms	Severity	Possible Triggers	Actions Taken

Symptom Tracker

Date	Symptoms	Severity	Possible Triggers	Actions Taken

Symptom Tracker

Date	Symptoms	Severity	Possible Triggers	Actions Taken

Symptom Tracker

Date	Symptoms	Severity	Possible Triggers	Actions Taken

Symptom Tracker

Date	Symptoms	Severity	Possible Triggers	Actions Taken

Symptom Tracker

Date	Symptoms	Severity	Possible Triggers	Actions Taken

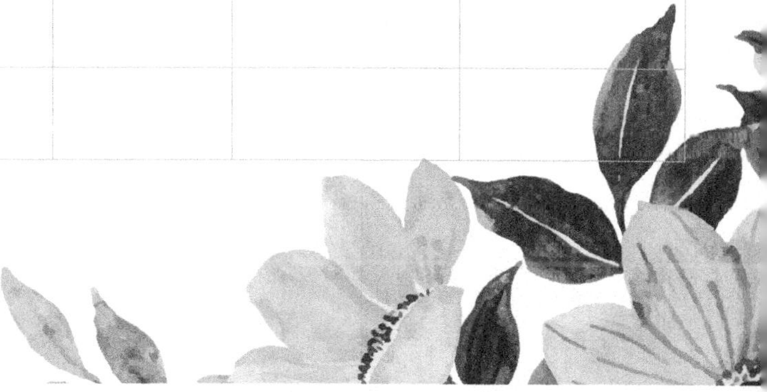

Symptom Tracker

Date	Symptoms	Severity	Possible Triggers	Actions Taken

Symptom Tracker

Date	Symptoms	Severity	Possible Triggers	Actions Taken

Symptom Tracker

Date	Symptoms	Severity	Possible Triggers	Actions Taken

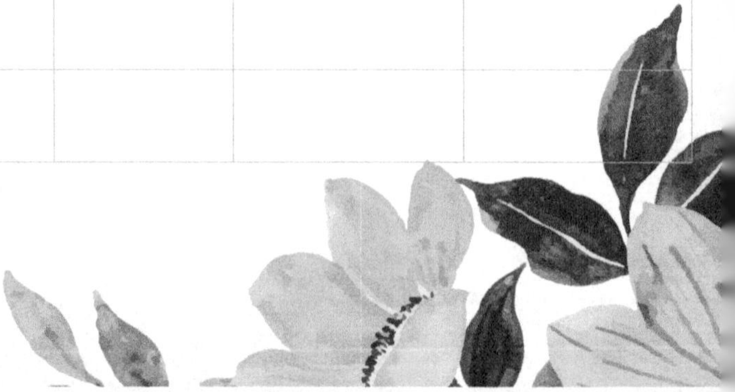

Symptom Tracker

Date	Symptoms	Severity	Possible Triggers	Actions Taken

Symptom Tracker

Date	Symptoms	Severity	Possible Triggers	Actions Taken

Symptom Tracker

Date	Symptoms	Severity	Possible Triggers	Actions Taken

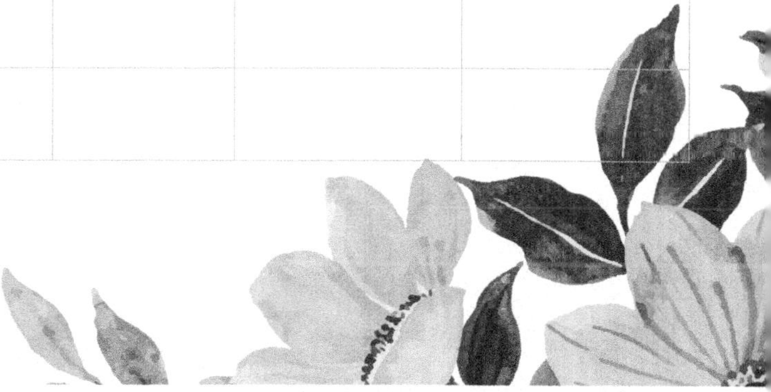

Symptom Tracker

Date	Symptoms	Severity	Possible Triggers	Actions Taken

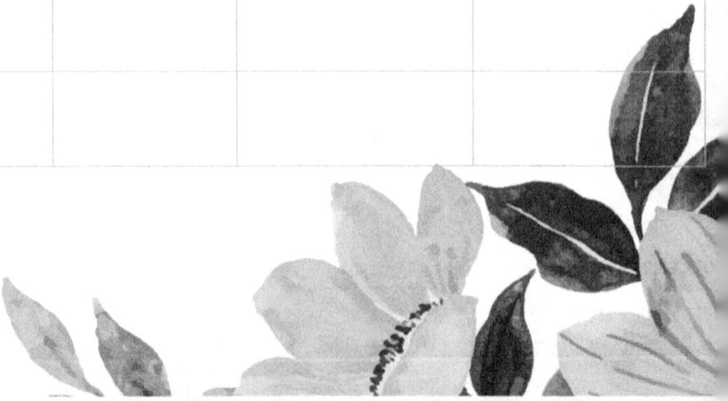

Symptom Tracker

Date	Symptoms	Severity	Possible Triggers	Actions Taken

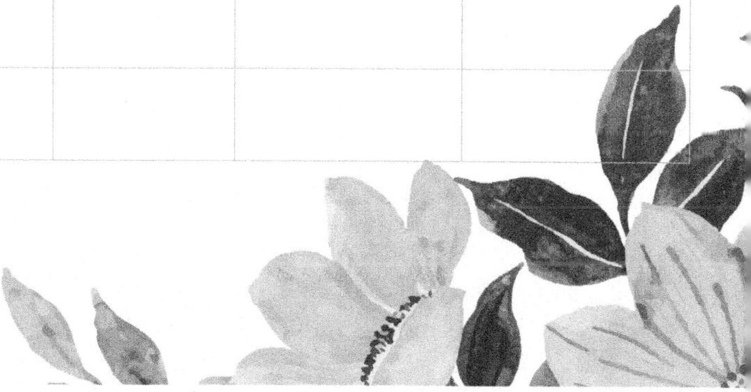

Symptom Tracker

Date	Symptoms	Severity	Possible Triggers	Actions Taken

Symptom Tracker

Date	Symptoms	Severity	Possible Triggers	Actions Taken

Symptom Tracker

Date	Symptoms	Severity	Possible Triggers	Actions Taken

Symptom Tracker

Date	Symptoms	Severity	Possible Triggers	Actions Taken

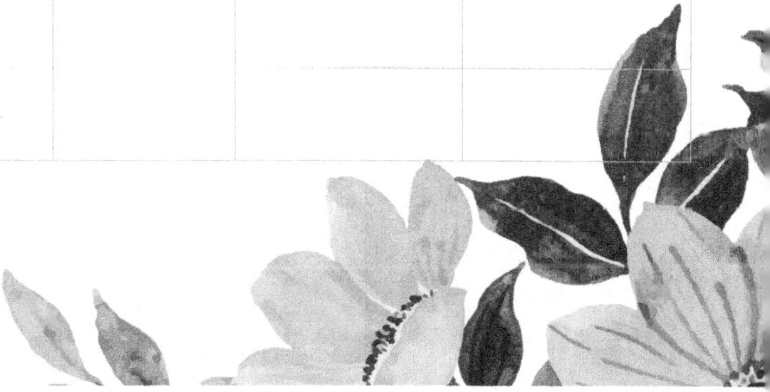

Symptom Tracker

Date	Symptoms	Severity	Possible Triggers	Actions Taken

Symptom Tracker

Date	Symptoms	Severity	Possible Triggers	Actions Taken

Symptom Tracker

Date	Symptoms	Severity	Possible Triggers	Actions Taken

Symptom Tracker

Date	Symptoms	Severity	Possible Triggers	Actions Taken

Symptom Tracker

Date	Symptoms	Severity	Possible Triggers	Actions Taken

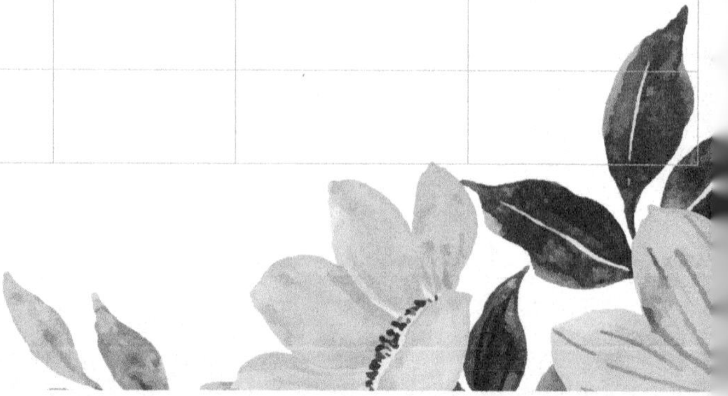

Symptom Tracker

Date	Symptoms	Severity	Possible Triggers	Actions Taken

Symptom Tracker

Date	Symptoms	Severity	Possible Triggers	Actions Taken

Symptom Tracker

Date	Symptoms	Severity	Possible Triggers	Actions Taken

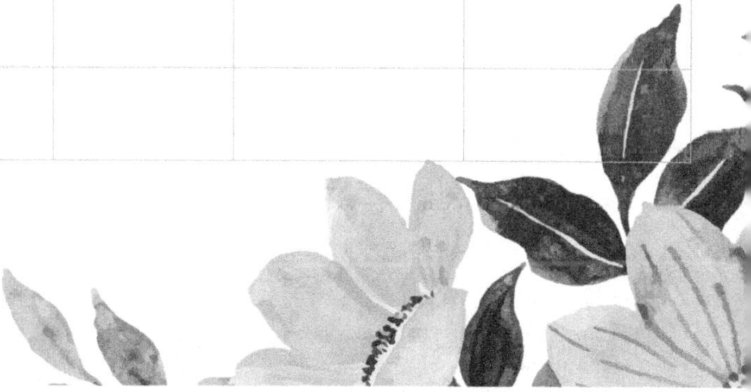

Symptom Tracker

Date	Symptoms	Severity	Possible Triggers	Actions Taken

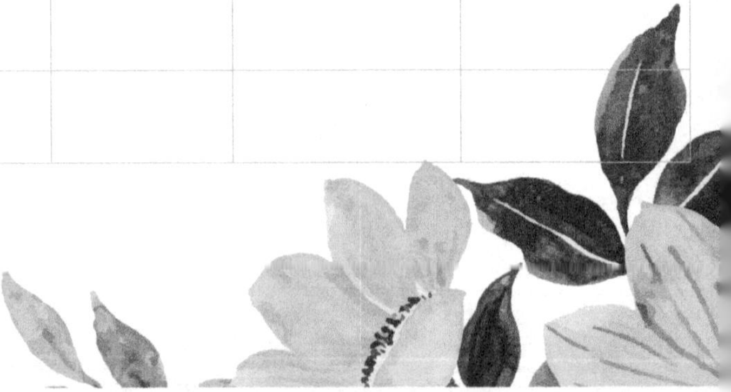

Symptom Tracker

Date	Symptoms	Severity	Possible Triggers	Actions Taken

Symptom Tracker

Date	Symptoms	Severity	Possible Triggers	Actions Taken

Symptom Tracker

Date	Symptoms	Severity	Possible Triggers	Actions Taken

Symptom Tracker

Date	Symptoms	Severity	Possible Triggers	Actions Taken

Symptom Tracker

Date	Symptoms	Severity	Possible Triggers	Actions Taken

Symptom Tracker

Date	Symptoms	Severity	Possible Triggers	Actions Taken

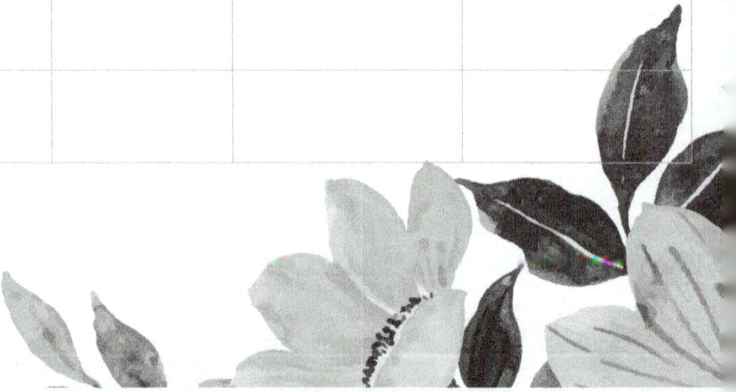

Symptom Tracker

Date	Symptoms	Severity	Possible Triggers	Actions Taken

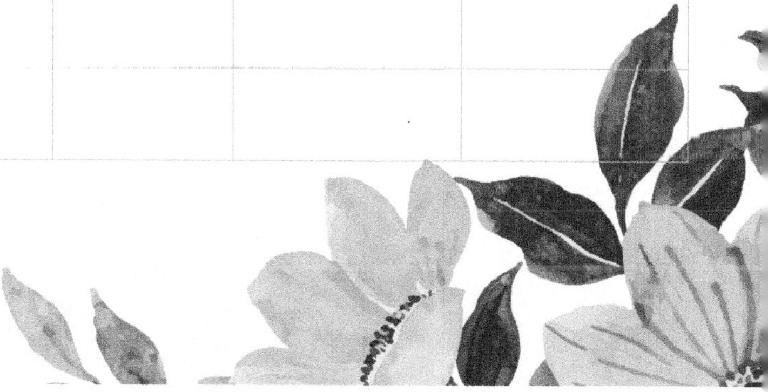

Symptom Tracker

Date	Symptoms	Severity	Possible Triggers	Actions Taken

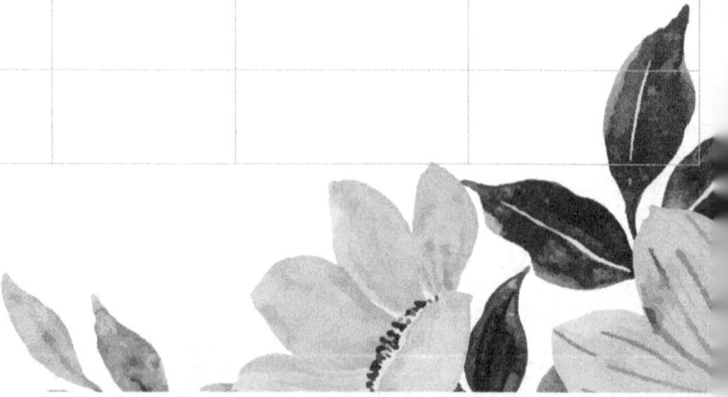

Symptom Tracker

Date	Symptoms	Severity	Possible Triggers	Actions Taken

Symptom Tracker

Date	Symptoms	Severity	Possible Triggers	Actions Taken

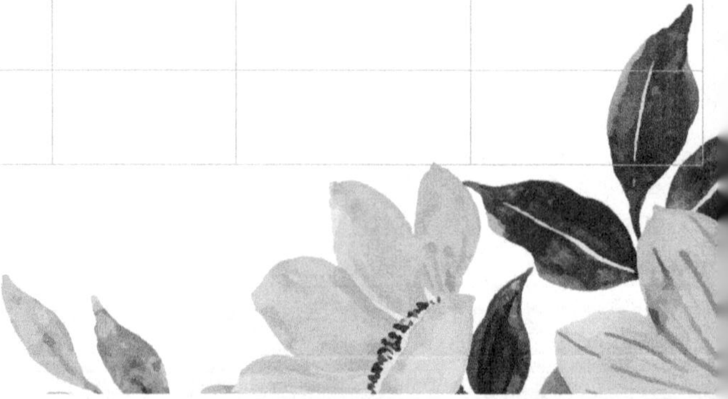

Symptom Tracker

Date	Symptoms	Severity	Possible Triggers	Actions Taken

Symptom Tracker

Date	Symptoms	Severity	Possible Triggers	Actions Taken

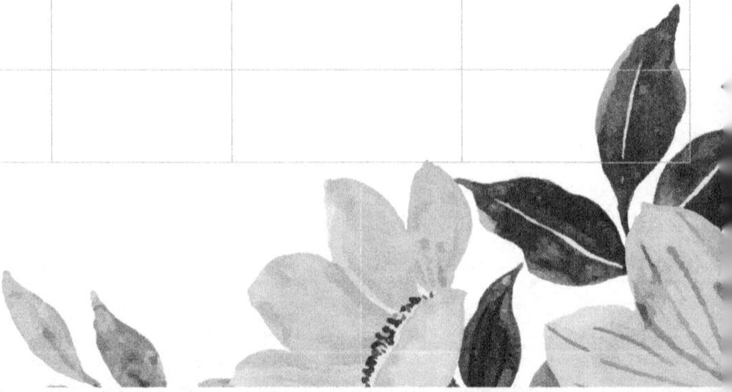

Symptom Tracker

Date	Symptoms	Severity	Possible Triggers	Actions Taken

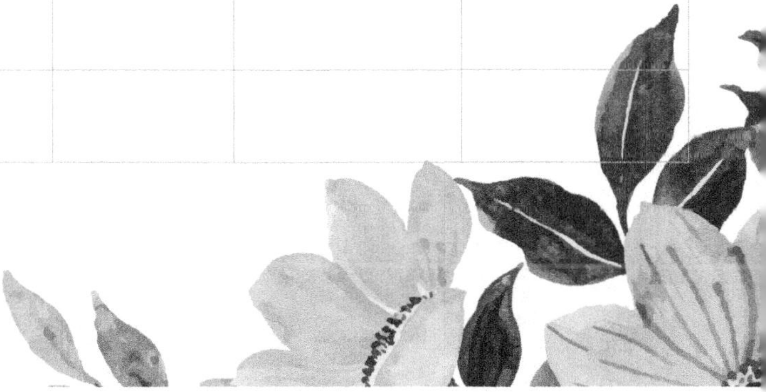

Symptom Tracker

Date	Symptoms	Severity	Possible Triggers	Actions Taken

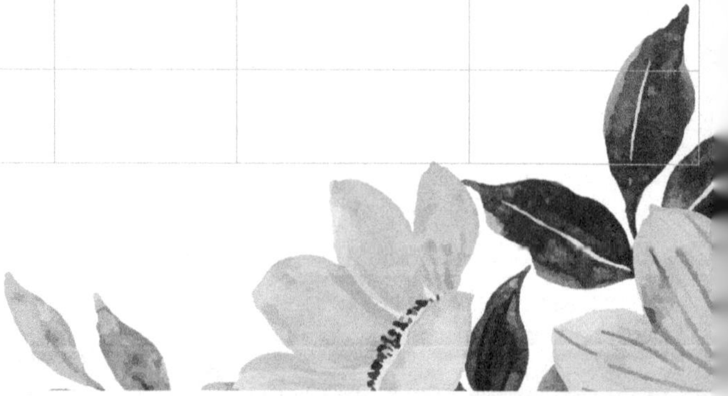

Symptom Tracker

Date	Symptoms	Severity	Possible Triggers	Actions Taken

Symptom Tracker

Date	Symptoms	Severity	Possible Triggers	Actions Taken

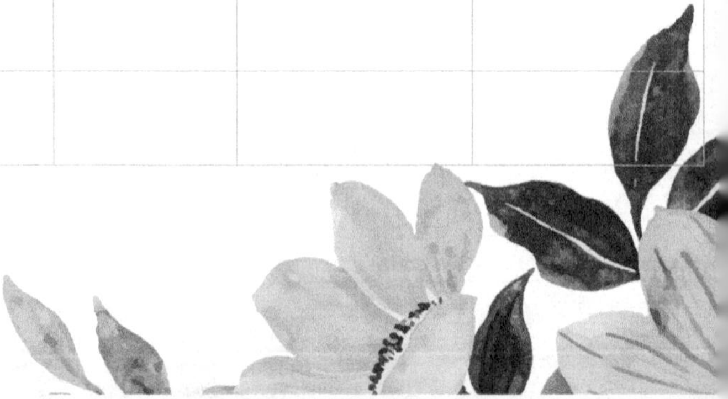

Symptom Tracker

Date	Symptoms	Severity	Possible Triggers	Actions Taken

Symptom Tracker

Date	Symptoms	Severity	Possible Triggers	Actions Taken

Symptom Tracker

Date	Symptoms	Severity	Possible Triggers	Actions Taken

Symptom Tracker

Date	Symptoms	Severity	Possible Triggers	Actions Taken

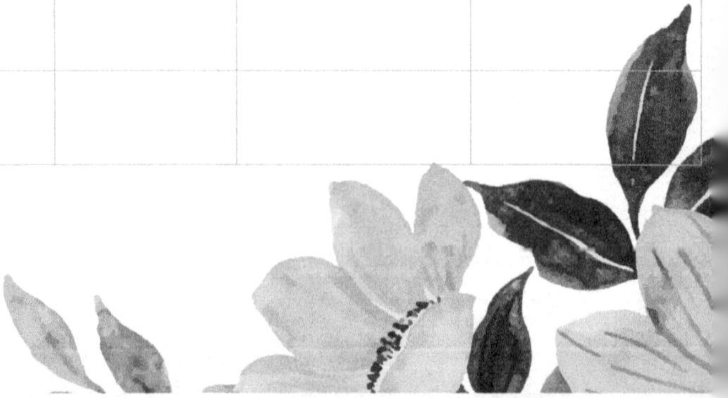

Symptom Tracker

Date	Symptoms	Severity	Possible Triggers	Actions Taken

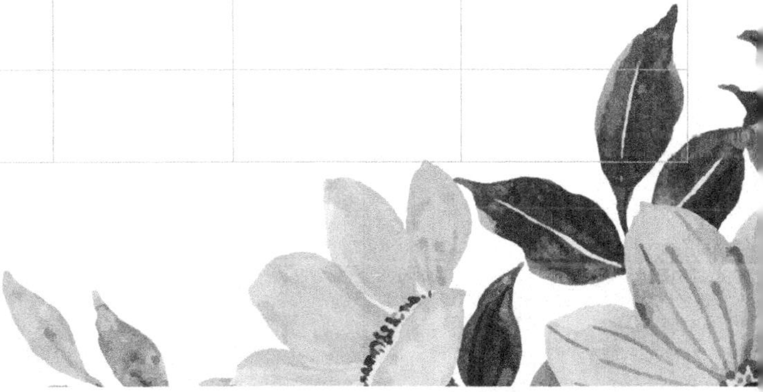

Symptom Tracker

Date	Symptoms	Severity	Possible Triggers	Actions Taken

Symptom Tracker

Date	Symptoms	Severity	Possible Triggers	Actions Taken

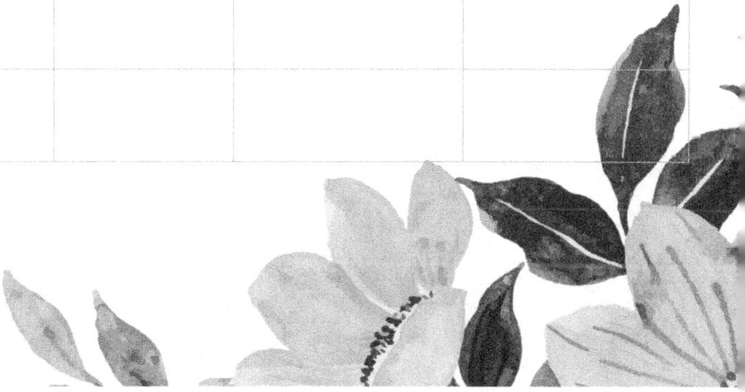

Symptom Tracker

Date	Symptoms	Severity	Possible Triggers	Actions Taken

Symptom Tracker

Date	Symptoms	Severity	Possible Triggers	Actions Taken

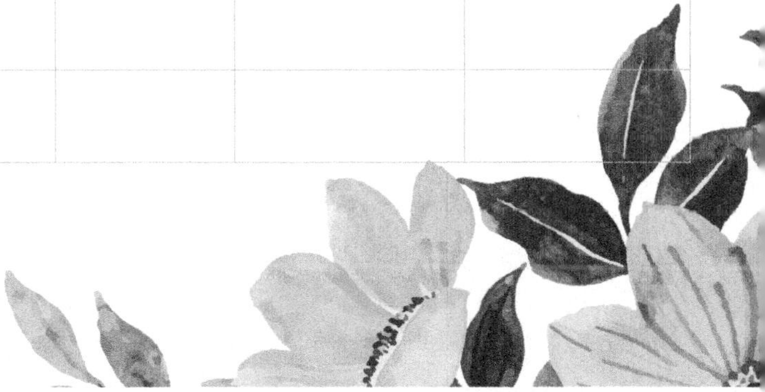

Symptom Tracker

Date	Symptoms	Severity	Possible Triggers	Actions Taken

Symptom Tracker

Date	Symptoms	Severity	Possible Triggers	Actions Taken

Symptom Tracker

Date	Symptoms	Severity	Possible Triggers	Actions Taken

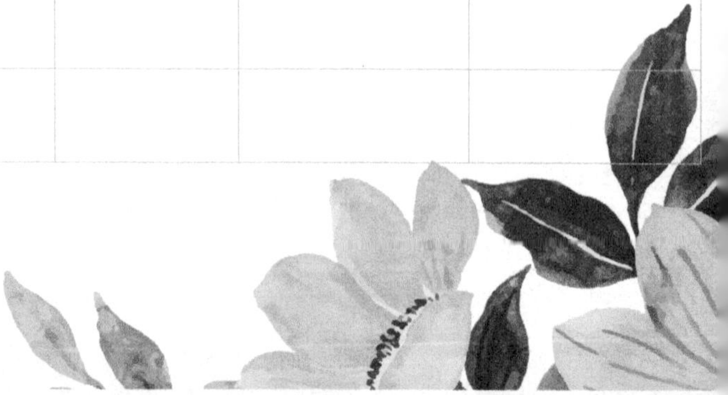

Symptom Tracker

Date	Symptoms	Severity	Possible Triggers	Actions Taken

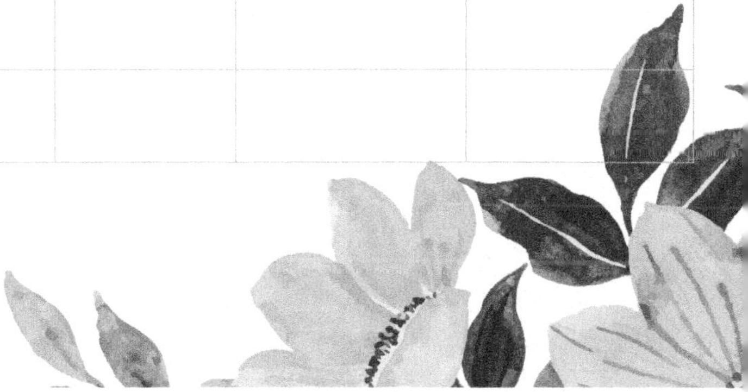

Symptom Tracker

Date	Symptoms	Severity	Possible Triggers	Actions Taken

Symptom Tracker

Date	Symptoms	Severity	Possible Triggers	Actions Taken

Symptom Tracker

Date	Symptoms	Severity	Possible Triggers	Actions Taken

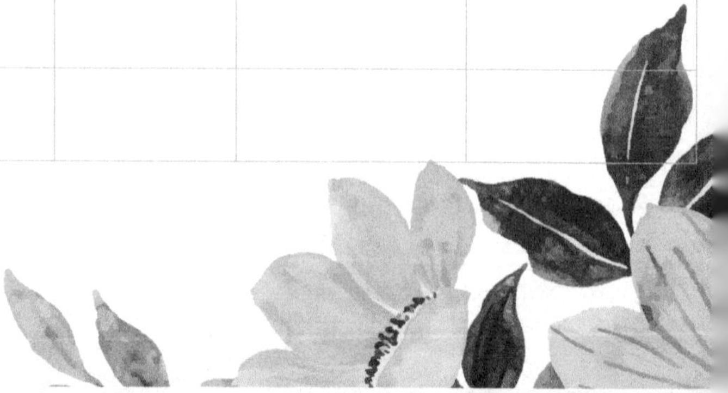

Symptom Tracker

Date	Symptoms	Severity	Possible Triggers	Actions Taken

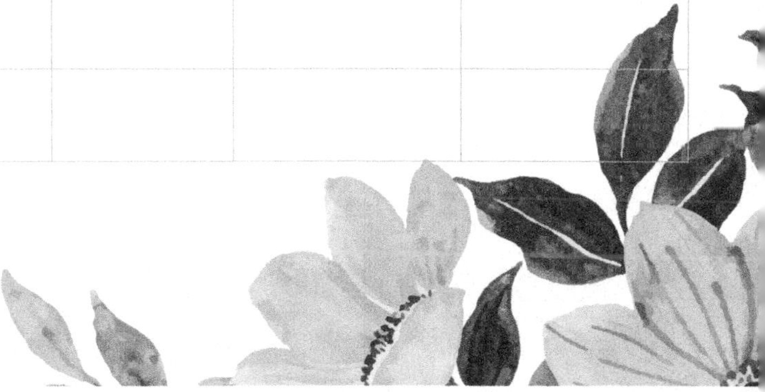

Symptom Tracker

Date	Symptoms	Severity	Possible Triggers	Actions Taken

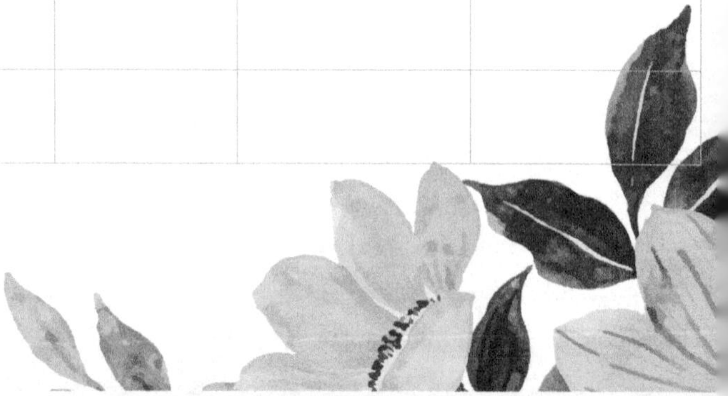

Made in the USA
Monee, IL
04 November 2026

67380877R00046